I0393384

"Wisdom only comes from Experience.
Knowledge and Experience
only come from
study and participation.
There is no shortcut."

The good news is
Everyone can study.
Everyone can gain experience.
Everyone can earn wisdom.

Audrey Friedman, RN

Copyright Information

Disclosures:
- I have no formal or financial relationship with Dr. Patricia Benner regarding my references to her nursing research 'Novice to Expert', I am just a big fan.
- I was a member of Sigma Theta Tau International in nursing school.

Also by Audrey Friedman, RN

Nursing Wit and Wisdom: Truths, Humor and Wisdom from the Stethescope to the Bedside, 2nd *edition*
Available at Amazon and Kindle
Bulk orders discount available. Please contact Audrey Friedman RN
At Audrey@FriedmanMedicalLegal.com

Nursing Wit and Wisdom
Blog: www.NursingWitAndWisdom.com

Nursing Wit and Wisdom at Facebook
www.Facebook.com/nursingwitandwisdom

Dedicated to:

This book is dedicated to my nursing orientees and students whom I have happily oriented, educated and mentored. It has been my pleasure and my honor to work with you and get to know you. You are all amazing Nightingales! Thank you for letting me use my Preceptor Project tools with you. I hope they have been helpful to you as a nurse and inspire you to use them yourselves to precept and mentor your colleagues and new nurses!

This book is also dedicated to the preceptors, nursing educators and bedside mentors that I have been privileged to work with and learn from their time, experience and wisdom.

It is because of their preparing and sharing fertile ground to ask questions, brainstorm ideas and situations, and seek opportunities that I have learned not only critical thinking nursing skills but been privileged of watching Nightingale genius and wisdom in action.

If I stand tall and am inspired, it is because I stand on your shoulders.
My hope is that I can inspire and support others as you have inspired and supported me.

Thank you!
Audrey

Are you ready to get your day started?

TABLE OF CONTENTS

A. Introduction

Dear Nightingales and Friends,

I am very excited to share with you the MAGIC PEARL I consider to be the cornerstone of my nursing preceptor toolbox.

The 3P's is a tool I have developed during my long, crazy curly, gray haired nursing career and my opportunities to precept all kinds of nurses: students, new graduates, experienced nurses and, specialties including oncology, bone marrow transplant and intensive care.

The 3Ps is part of a bigger project I am calling "THE PRECEPTOR PROJECT" and part of the overall vision of my nursing project NURSING WIT AND WISDOM. I will tell you more about both, in a little bit, I promise.

One of nursing's finest core values and skills is to be able to educate patients, families, communities, physicians, students, and each other. It doesn't matter whether you are teaching a patient or family member about a medication, how to do a tube feeding or lecturing in a hall of students... A nurse is always an educator!

What makes a nurse so exquisitely suited to precepting? The Nursing Process! These are tools you already know and can be used in perfect format to precepting!

In my personal experience, The 3Ps, my favorite precepting pearl – works in every situation, with every kind of student and can fix MOST precepting problems.

Sounds impossible?

Not so! Over my precepting experience, I have toned and honed and tweaked and dusted and trialed The 3Ps in every teaching and precepting experience with which I have been involved.

Precepting came slowly. It started with offering to help other nurses. Then being a mentor to new nurses, then starting to precept. I took the offered precepting classes. As time went on, I developed my own way of teaching – as all of us do.

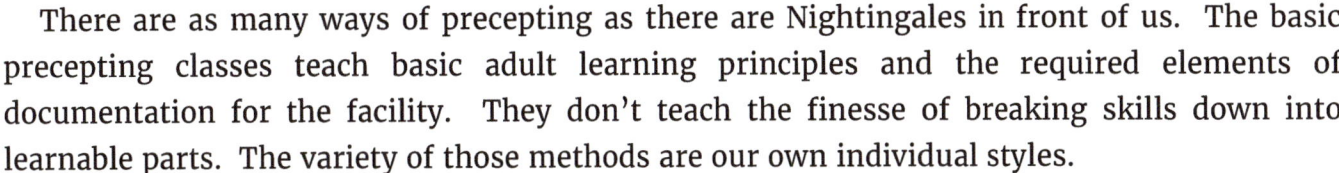

There are as many ways of precepting as there are Nightingales in front of us. The basic precepting classes teach basic adult learning principles and the required elements of documentation for the facility. They don't teach the finesse of breaking skills down into learnable parts. The variety of those methods are our own individual styles.

Through the years of precepting, I read books on mentoring, coaching techniques, tried out different techniques and developed my own. Eventually, the pieces came together into a style I used repeatedly in a method from front to back that I could call my own preceptor method.

I was able to test this method with various nurses in different situations. When I was asked to troubleshoot precepting experiences for a few new nurses, these were great opportunities to further develop The 3Ps. Every single nurse that I precepted using The 3Ps succeeded in graduating orientation. Every single nurse who was oriented using my preceptor program succeeded in becoming successful nursing staff, or using their skills as an independent practitioner. No one quit a job prematurely. No one was fired.

The unexpected part was how happy they were at the end of their orientation. They went from scared and fearful of their job, to happy and confident. All bullying from other nurses stopped. And to my humble joyful surprise, they often gifted me with cards and presents.

And the pearl that I call my magic key? The 3Ps!

I have found it gives new preceptors a quick, easy tool to teach both intellectual and didactic clinical experiences.

I have found it helps experienced nurses give pinpoint focus to their clinical issues quickly and perfectly.

In my experience with these nurses, I have found The 3Ps to be 100% successful in turning around confusion, overwhelm and despair that they are not capable of working in a unit.

It gives burned out preceptors a way to find joy again in precepting.

It stops bullying in precepting. It creates stronger clinical nurses. And it creates stronger nursing teams.

I hope you will see the same opportunities in improving nursing precepting that I have found with using 'The 3Ps' in your nursing,
    precepting and mentoring experiences.

I am excited to help you. I want to help you enjoy orientation. I want to help you enjoy precepting. I want to help you enjoy nursing.

That is what my vision for my project 'Nursing Wit and Wisdom' is all about:

> *"Helping nurses and nursing students find ways to stay excited about nursing*
> *and understand their unique position to influence others so that they can be inspired*
> *about the impact they can make*
> *on their patients, families, community and each other."*

Thank you, Nightingales, – for sharing your expertise, time and energy and excitement for nursing with others when you precept.
    You are so appreciated!

Inspire and Be Inspired Nightingales!
Audrey Friedman, RN,

B. About Audrey Friedman RN

Dear Nightingales and Friends,

When I read a book, the first thing I always read first – even before I read, borrow or buy the book – is WHO wrote it and WHO are they? So, let me share a little of my story with you...

I have been a registered nurse RN for 30+ years. I initially graduated a diploma nursing school in 1986 at Lutheran General Deaconess Hospital Nursing School, in Park Ridge, Illinois. At the time, it was a diploma school and adjacent to the hospital. This was very convenient, since we all felt like we lived there... school in the morning, clinicals in the afternoon and worked as CNAs in the hospital in the evenings.

I came to that school after two and a half years in the nursing program at Bradley University in Peoria, Illinois. I loved both schools, and fate gave me an opportunity to experience both BSN and Diploma programs, which ultimately helped both my clinical practice and my teaching and precepting experiences.

This, by the way, was in the era of white uniforms and nursing caps. I always wanted to be a nurse. I was that little girl who read Florence Nightingale and Clara Barton books, perused pictures of nursing uniforms and caps and could be found at the bedroom mirror, practicing the best ways to pin on my cap. My heart still flutters at the site of a white cap. Yes, yes... I am one of those. I love being *an old white cap*. ☺

After graduating from Lutheran General, I moved to Denver, Colorado and started my first nursing job in NICU III. I completed my BSN at Regis University in Denver, Colorado.

In my career, I have worked in NICU III, Research, oncology research, oncology, oncology for travel nursing, bone marrow transplant, intensive care, cardiology, education, case management and legal nurse consulting. I have done nursing mentoring and volunteer community health talks. I have worked full time hospital (days and mostly nights), office clinic, lawyer's office and home office. I have worked all kinds of shifts.

And here, at the 30-year mark – I still love nursing. I still love bedside nursing – the connection with the patient and their family – in whatever form that takes – inpatient, clinic, telephone, community.

I hope you do too. And if not, I hope I can help you find your way to your *Happy Place* in nursing.

Inspire and Be Inspired, Nightingales!

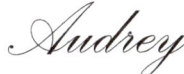

C. About Precepting

What is precepting? Merriam-Webster's dictionary defines **_"preceptor" as: "teacher or tutor"._**

There is an enormous scholarly library in nursing research attentive to multiple layers of precepting issues.

A quick internet response to "nursing preceptors" returns thousands of articles on research on topics including:

1. Education of preceptor
2. Retention of preceptors
3. Effect of preceptors on retention of new nurses
4. Effect of preceptors on quality of skills of new nurses
5. Differences of precepting students, new nurses and experienced nurses
6. Types of preceptor personalities
7. Preceptor burnout
8. The social theories of precepting and orientation that crossover between other professional environments: attorneys, teachers, physicians, military, retail, social work, etc., etc., etc.

I am glad to see more research and activity geared toward the preceptor themselves. For many years, the only education preceptors received were two topics:

1. Adult learning styles
2. Standard of care and facility regulatory requirements

I call this **"Level I Preceptor Education"**.

We are going to work on what I call, _"Level II Preceptor Orientation":_
1. Specific Preceptor Education with teaching skills and specific tools
2. Designing a unit specific orientation (this part we'll do in The Preceptor Project)

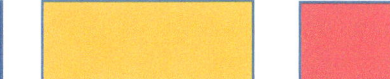

I truly believe, by my 30 years of experience, as a nurse in many different roles: student, staff, charge, case manager, care coordinator, preceptor, educator, orientation development, mentor and legal nurse that...

- *Precepting is a multi-factorial responsibility and activity that uses various social roles including teacher, hostess, mentor, parent and friend, to achieve success in 3 BASIC AREAS of work success:*

  - **KNOWLEDGE:** using basic and advanced conceptual information that provides the fundamental knowledge required to engage in multidimensional critical thinking related to patient care issues, nursing interventions and assessments;
  - **TASKS**: assessing basic nursing skills and providing education, experience and opportunity to progress competence and advanced clinical and technical skill set;
  - **SOCIALIZATION:** assisting, encouraging and engaging new staff into social acceptance into a new group process. Basically, you are assisting the social introduction and acceptance of not only the individual as a clinical provider to patients and families, but also to the existing family team and the relative units and departments that interact with your family team.

The WHO, WHAT, WHERE, WHEN, WHY and HOW you are asking yourself now...
You already know!

Yes, yes, you do!

You know this skill inside and out!

You have spent years learning it, practicing it and incorporating it into your very nursing soul until it aligns with the way you breathe and you do it most of the time without even thinking about it!

Have you guessed what it is?

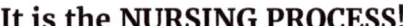

It is the NURSING PROCESS!
   a. Assessment: collecting and analyzing data
   b. Diagnosing: your clinical judgement regarding actual or potential needs
   c. Planning Outcomes: setting measurable short and long term goals
   d. Implementation: creating action of steps that accomplish agreed goals
   e. Evaluating: re-assessing the effectiveness of the outcome of the steps in relation to the goals from the identified original needs and deciding if there is success or a need to adjust outcome goals and/or steps to accomplish success.

Nightingales, Remember...

You do this every day.

In some cases, intuitively.

In some cases, as a team care management presentation to brainstorm a plan of care as a team.

In some cases, as a preceptor, charge nurse, colleague or mentor, to breakdown a complex care situation into identifiable care differentials and a treatment plan that you will implement, then evaluate and report effectiveness to the physician or care team.

So, bring that amazing skill with you –

Because we are going to learn how to use it in a fantastic, fun and successful way for precepting!

D. My Favorite Research Tool

My favorite nursing theorist and teaching tool is from Dr. Patricia Benner and her theory on clinical competence in her book: "From Novice to Expert: Excellence and Power in Clinic Nursing Practice" (1982). If you are a preceptor or wanting to be on, I highly recommend you get this book – and read it!

While my book is not a tutorial on her theory, I hope you have had the pleasure of hearing it or reading it somewhere in nursing school or in clinical practice.

Here is the link to her theory at www.nursing-theory.org:
http://www.nursing-theory.org/theories-and-models/from-novice-to-expert.php

Dr. Benner builds her theory on the research of knowledge acquisition by The Dreyfus Model of Skill Acquisition, a learning theory based from observations of how chess players and the military, to discover how people learn, using observations and experiences to build skills.

Dr. Benner created five stages of learning to describe how nursing education, observation and experience cumulate from being a nursing student to an expert through skill competence and expertise.

> ### The 5 Stages of Benner's Novice to Expert include:
> **Stage 1: Novice**
> **Stage 2: Advanced Beginner**
> **Stage 3: Competent**
> **Stage 4: Proficient**
> **Stage 5: Expert**

What I really love about Benner's Novice to Expert is that Dr. Benner describes in detail how each year of experience ties in to cognitive thinking and processing and how that is demonstrated in skill ability.

It also gave me a HUGE insight about my precepting. Once I understood where my orientee or student was, in their learning curve, per Benner's Novice to Expert, I could easily pare my teaching style and level expertise to match their understanding. And, Benner's gave me some insight about ways to teach each level.

For example – Novice learners, per Benner, are very task oriented. Meds on time. They can struggle understanding priorities if they interfere with getting a task done on time.

This can also be a huge insight as a preceptor when I find a nurse is struggling with the plan of care for the day.

I can break it down into tasks, priorities, plans and panic areas.

Dr. Benner is one of many research studies, tools, and references for nursing research related to nursing education. I know I am an academic geek – my inner academic geek and my inner Nightingale Preceptor Mama loves to read nursing research especially when it relates to nursing orientation, the how, why, resources, retention, transition, etc.

But there isn't a lot related to teaching us, the preceptor specific tools and skills.

There is a great program I took with Sigma Theta Tau International and the International Council of Nurses, called, "Coaching in Nursing". Coaching skills are an absolute and underused positive force in precepting! You can find it at this link at Nursing Knowledge International:

https://www.nursingknowledge.org/coaching-in-nursing-online-course.html

Many clinical facilities, especially hospitals have worked very hard to determine the most proficient way to orient nursing staff to their units and facilities.

Orientation is different in every situation, clinical specialty, the level of acuity in a unit, hospital or facility, culture of population and culture of nurses. You name it, it will be a factor in orienting new nursing staff.

There is a lot of great research stuff out there by your colleagues!

GET OUT THERE AND READ IT! USE IT!

CREATE YOUR OWN IDEAS!

MAKE RESEARCH OF YOUR OWN!

I hope these tools will help inspire you to create tools of your own!

Write them down. Test them. Teach them. Share them.

Will you be the next nursing research article I read about?

I HOPE SO!

E. How I created The 3Ps

How DID I create The 3Ps?

There wasn't really a MOMENT. There were m.o.m.e.n.t.s.

There were moments I didn't understand something and I had to think of how to break it down, understand it, digest it and put it back together in a way I could use again and again and I needed help. For example:

a. One of my favorite preceptors in ICU was a charge nurse, whom I am convinced had secret powers. She had the ability to always be right where you needed her even without asking. I would be ready to turn and go find her, and instead I would turn and almost walk right into her. One night, I was standing at the door to my patient's room and was watching the cardiac monitor while I trying to put some clinical pieces together. I wasn't understanding how the cardiac rhythms were matching the changes in status I was seeing. Next thing I know, she was standing right next to me and asked me what I was trying to figure out. Then she said to me, "just talk it out loud. Talk everything you are thinking about, out loud. There is no right or wrong. Let me hear how you are thinking about it". So, I started to go through all the pieces. In a moment, she picked up on the exact problem and could teach me the cause and effect of the cardiac rhythms I was seeing. It was helpful, insightful, comforting, inspiring and supportive. All by standing quietly next to me and listening. This was an inspiration of a great preceptor/mentor.

b. I had another preceptor in ICU who came to me as I was at the desk and had my papers out – my report sheet, my medication papers, my book references and the computer open to the patient record. I was focused on diligently trying to figure out something I did not understand about the case and trying to find *what* I didn't understand. My preceptor asked what I was doing, and I explained that I was confused about some issue and was trying to figure it out. She said to me, "Don't worry, I know you got this!" Her response, I think was meant to be supportive and encouraging, but instead I found it dismissive and, I started getting frustrated even just by getting stuck.

So, I stopped. I stepped back and asked myself, "What AREA do you think you are stuck at: Physiology? Pathophysiology? Medication? Labs? Test Results? Procedure? Once I could pick the one place I was confused about, I went directly to that area, found the question and then took that specific question to my preceptor. This was my inspiration of how an orientee can use or create a teaching tool that can help themselves and use their preceptor for their expertise in clinical expertise even if they are not the greatest preceptor.

Sometimes great Nightingales are experts clinically and have a hard time sharing their knowledge in pieces, steps and pathways that encourage learning. It doesn't make them less of an expert. But it can be frustrating. The 3P tools can also help nurses teach themselves.

c. Then there are nurses I have worked with in my long career that I could honestly call my special Nightingales angels. They are nurses I worked with that were so amazing in their expertise in clinical practice, precepting, mentoring and leadership that I would involuntarily stop, frozen from what I was doing and watch and listen to whatever they were doing. The room could be on fire, with flames spitting everywhere and people running around like chaos. They would enter, look around and say, "Well, what have we got here?", calm and collected like they were choosing tea in a cake shop. Immediately, a calm and organization would come over the room when they were there.

What was it that I found so amazing about these Nightingales? It was two things:

a. They listened. They didn't judge my question or me. They always praised my question or my inquiry.

b. They could see what I was trying to get to and could break the question down into pieces and explain each section so that in the end, I could put the pieces back together on my own, and they would let me get there.

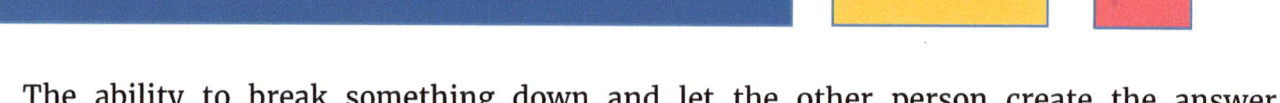

The ability to break something down and let the other person create the answer for themselves, I think, was the beginning of The 3Ps .

The 3Ps helped me break down the ENTIRE SHIFT, and help my student create it in a way they could understand and control (considering the fact we work in an environment that is not controllable!)

There are many Nightingales I admire for this trait... and how they mentor other Nightingales. Some are crunchy and tough to approach and some are soft, snuggly and motherly. Each one has something special that makes them sought after, appreciated and respected. They deserve every word, every thank you and every appreciation we say and don't say!

So, reach out and give a well-deserved 'Thank you!' to your own special Nightingale mentor!

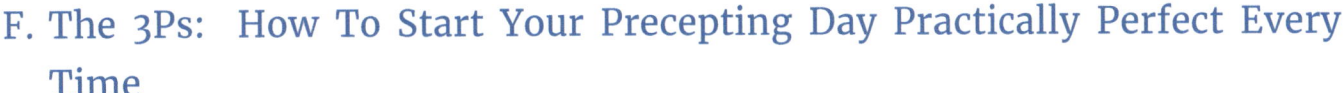

F. The 3Ps: How To Start Your Precepting Day Practically Perfect Every Time

The goal of a lot of teaching techniques is to be able to break down complex clinical concepts into tiny bits that are easily understandable and then reconnect them back to the full concept that can be applied to clinical practice.

I believe preceptors should be prepared to be able to teach a concept of skill 5 different ways. Each learner comes from different places: language, nursing experiences, level of medical complexity, experience as a nursing assistant, military medic, EMT, paramedic and nursing school. Nursing schools may currently be focused on bachelors or associate, but at one time there were also diploma schools as well. Each type of school teaches the same concept but can vary in teacher clinical experience and creativity in applying teaching techniques.

So basically, the experience of the orientee in front of you can be ANYTHING!

Are you prepared for ANYTHING?

You can be.

The 3Ps are all we need to get a running, prepared, organized start to your shift.

My personal favorite place to start a new orientee is to use The 3Ps as our daily preparation.

First, let me explain how The 3Ps can be your *secret pearl* to be able to handle any orientee experience.

If you are already a preceptor or, an experienced nurse, remember... you may already do this intuitively and automatically, because of your experience. The 3Ps tool will help you break down your experienced intuition into teachable steps for your student or orientee.

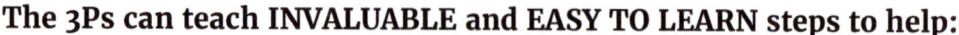

The 3Ps can teach INVALUABLE and EASY TO LEARN steps to help:

1. REVIEW AND PLAN your entire shift
2. To PROBLEM SOLVE a clinical issue
3. Understand the CLINICAL ISSUES
4. Be able to PRIORITIZE clinical issues
5. Be PREPARED for when the clinical situation CHANGES
6. Be able to REACT FASTER to patient needs, clinical changes and clinical emergencies

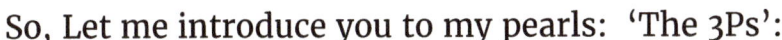

So, Let me introduce you to my pearls: 'The 3Ps':

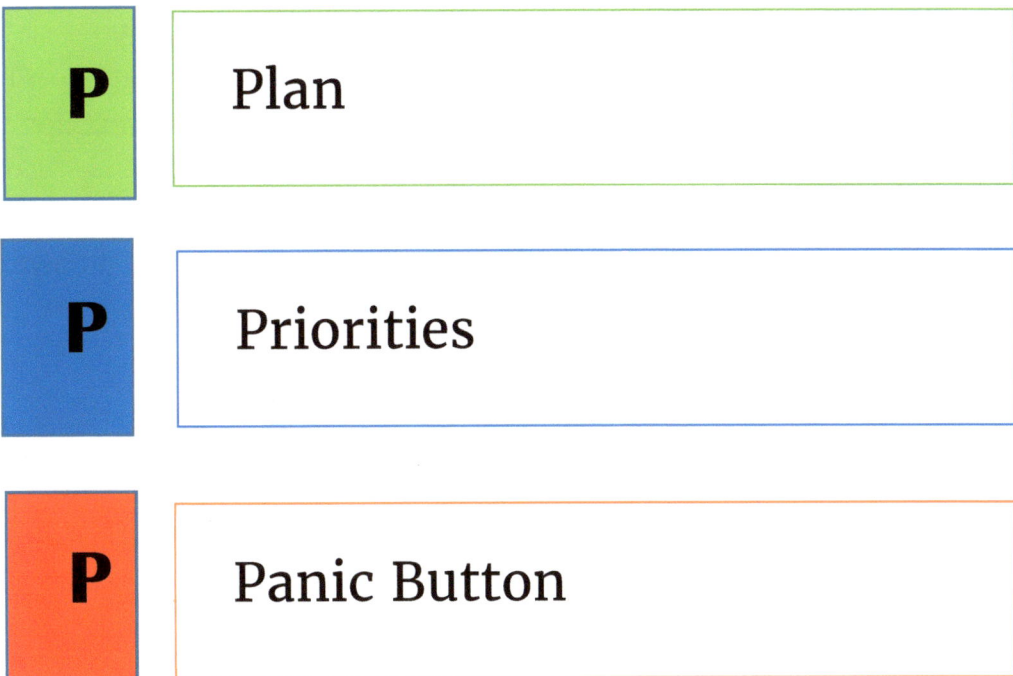

Let's go over each of them in a little more detail.

My daily goal is to have the orientee review all 3Ps after report, given some time, and BEFORE we start seeing patients.

They will be tempted to run, dash, sprint – and get started. I have had to pull a few back from a sprint to review The 3Ps.

The sprint out of report can be appropriate if your patient is in trouble, of course. Otherwise, it is more likely that it is due to fear and overwhelm – so much to do and unsure where to start.

Show them they can do it organized, purposeful and calmly – with The 3Ps .

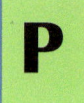 **P** **Plan**

THE PLAN:

a. Start with this piece at the beginning of your day
b. This is the list of 1000 things to do you heard in Report (Shift Report, Admission Report, Transfer Report or the mob that met you at the door when you came in the office
c. You are gathering all the information you need, here.
d. Don't worry about getting it all done. Just write it down.
e. Go to the next step: P/Priorities

The idea behind THE PLAN is that so often students, new nurses or nurses new to new clinical environments get very overwhelmed with the amount of information given during report.

Nurses going off shift are trying earnestly to give every important detail of what happened during their shift and what needs to be done in just a few minutes of tape-recorded or live in-person report. The on-coming nurse tries to write every detail given during report and often lose their organization even if they are using a designed report sheet.

And if that patient just arrived or is in the middle of decompensating clinically and procedures are in progress, there is often no organization to the report at all. It is just a lot of information thrown out to try to convey everything that is happening.

That is normal. We work with sick and very sick people. We can't turn off the conveyor belt for report.

What we CAN do is systematically train and practice and train some more – to learn how to use The 3Ps and easily categorize and prioritize where to start.

As a seasoned nurse, you can listen to report and easily pick out where to start. I know some nurses that don't even write report.

We all know our favorite expert nurses who can listen to report at the desk or listen to report at the bedside during a chaotic admission or resuscitation and process it all in a blink of an eye and seem to calmly have it all handled when the rest of the world has been running around like their shoes are on fire! They listen to report and know exactly where to start. That takes time, practice and experience. Something a new nurse doesn't have – yet.

Giving them access to great tools is the perfect way to help them train, learn, practice and gain experience. In time, their organizational ability will get stronger – just like yours did.

Priorities

THE PRIORITIES:

    a. Out of the 1000 Things To Do you identified in The Plan, now, choose the TOP 3-5 things that MUST be done as a CLINICAL PRIORITY for your shift or the time you have left with the patient or, your office

    b. Start with the CLINICAL PRIORITY

PRIORITIES is the ability to take in the 1000 things the reporting nurse is telling you and easily reach in to the pile and pick out the top 3-5 things that have *CLINICAL IMPORTANCE OR URGENCY* over everything else.

A new nurse can struggle finding priority when tasks, and 'tasks on time' can seem like the priority. This is due to nursing school's training them about the importance of promptness. Remember, per Benner's Novice to Expert, Novices are very task oriented and can often prioritize timed tasks over anything else. And they can easily feel like they are doing something wrong if something is late. And timeliness IS IMPORTANT – or we all would be doing 24 hour shifts just to get our 12-hour work done.

However, the ability to PRIORITIZE for CLINICAL IMPORTANCE OR URGENCY is an invaluable skill that can:

1. **Prevent problems**
2. **Minimize decompensation of a patient**
3. **Provide opportunities for multi-tasking**

The **KEY** is to be able to explain

WHAT IS CLINICAL IMPORTANCE
AND URGENCY
IN YOUR CLINICAL SPECIALTY.

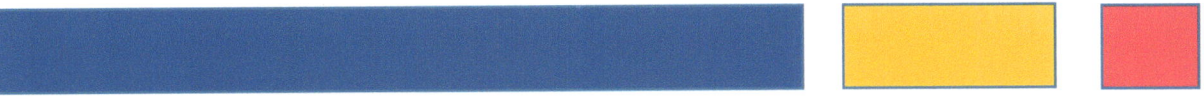

Use this KEY of Clinical Importance and Urgency to break down the concept of PRIORITIES into pieces to your orientee.

1. Clearly, the ABC's of airway, breathing and circulation come first.
2. Next, are you on a surgical floor, an oncology floor, a pediatric floor, an intensive care floor? Are you in a clinic?
3. What are the clinical priorities with your patient population?
4. With their diagnoses?
5. With their procedures?

As you gain experience, you may think it is very easy to prioritize your plan of care for the day. Yes, it does get easier. And soon, it becomes second nature and you can do it without much forethought.

Panic Button

THE PANIC BUTTON:

1. What is the WORST thing that could happen to this patient today?
2. How would you recognize it?
3. What would you do about it?
4. What RESOURCES would you need? Know where they are or pull them together NOW.
5. Who could you ALERT to be on watch with you?

Remember, developing the ability to prioritize for CLINICAL IMPORTANCE OR URGENCY is an invaluable skill that can not only strategize PRIORITIES, but can be a key to:
   a. Prevent problems
   b. Minimize decompensation of a patient
   c. Provide opportunities for multi-tasking

So, in using this theory, let's take a moment and think of THE WORST thing that could happen to your patient today. Of course, it will vary by what specialty unit you are on. That part does not matter.

Think of it this way...
What would make you drop what you are doing and leave your food or run from the bathroom?
That is panic!
AAAAAhhhhhhgggggghhhhhhh!!!!!!

What DOES matter is that thinking of the WORST thing DOES TWO THINGS:
   It helps the student THINK PATIENT CARE ALL THE WAY THROUGH...
   1. "If this happens, then what?
   2. "If this happens, then what?
   3. "If this happens, then what?

Now... they have already started to ANTICIPATE WHAT TO DO.

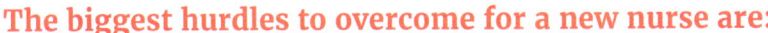

The biggest hurdles to overcome for a new nurse are:

1. FEAR of not knowing what to do
2. STUN – the moment fear becomes immobility

We have all seen – or been – the orientee that gets so overwhelmed in a decompensating situation that they can't initiate action, they can barely follow direction and sometimes we find them/ourselves in the corner watching it all go by.   OK if you have a team with you that can take over. Not great if you are the only one in the patient's room.

There is ALWAYS something even a new nurse can do. Reassure them that there are things they already know how to do: place oxygen, get vital signs, hang normal saline intravenous fluids, start writing a timeline, get supplies... These are things they do all day, every day, every shift. And they are perfect places to start and let them become accustomed to chaos.

There ARE many things on your unit they already know how to do and can do them in an emergency, while they are learning to do more, and the more experienced nurses are jumping in.

The best thing that can help a STUNNED nurse snap out of it, is to be given something to do.

1. Write down vitals
2. Write down everything that is happening
3. Hang IV Normal Saline
4. Get more bags of normal saline

As they get more experienced and you see less stun and more focus and initiative, you can involve them in decision making. But the first step is to BREAK THE STUN.

As the preceptor, with your superpower Nightingale extra senses, you have already assessed the situation and know 47 things that could go wrong – even before report is over. So start asking questions...

1. What happens if you run out of your Levophed drip?
2. What happens if the Tylenol doesn't bring down the fever?
3. What happens if the valium doesn't last 3 hours?
4. What happens if...
5. What are your 47 questions?

Assess your orientee for learning readiness. At the beginning, you WILL NEED TO MAKE extra time to ask questions, give resources and allow conversation.

Later, you will be able to just shoot the questions off at any moment.

Take your new nurse to crash situations. If there are people to spare, the two of you can stand in the back and you can narrate the situation and ask questions. That is a good way to start, if you can, because there is a lot to see and a lot to talk about.

While you are asking, "What's next?", "Why are they hanging that?", "Why are they getting an arterial line ready?" … and answering some of the questions, eventually, they will be able to have a broader view of the room and start picking up what is going on.
Ask the questions – WHO, WHAT, WHY, WHEN, WHERE, HOW and WHAT IF?

Talk it through. Let them listen to you talk it through. Let them hear your wisdom to who, what, why, when, how, what if and... not on my shift!!

The PANIC BUTTON is a perfect learning tool to progress the nurses' learning to a whole new level THAT CAN INCLUDE ANTICIPATION.

They may not get the entire scope of what you are observing and where you are leading them in the question and conversation.

But the more you open the skylight and look up, look past, look through...

1. They will start ANTICIPATING in their care
2. They will know that questions, and conversation and brainstorming together creates learning, creates experiences and creates a fantabulousistic team!

Walk towards the panic to succeed! Don't run from it!

So, get out there and create some Panic!

G. Handy Dandy Nightingale Tips

1. **There is NO SHORTCUT to learning and practice. Use The 3Ps EVERY SHIFT AND EVERY DAY BEFORE you go into a patients' room. Use them to answer questions. Use them to mentor other nurses. Make your day impossible to start without The 3Ps!**
   1. It will help you evaluate their knowledge, skills and critical thinking and where the holes are,
   2. From there, YOU can adjust YOUR teaching needs for the day,
   3. It will help YOU know they are prepared

2. **Realize that different units and kinds of nursing groups need to organize differently.** Patient populations, staffing, daily report, unit routines are all different. No unit, office, clinic, home care or hospice is the same. The last place I tweaked and used The 3Ps was in the ICU. However, they were inspired and designed in NICU, on an oncology floor, drafted and written in Bone Marrow Transplant and polished in ICU. I have used them on floor staff, ICU staff and nursing students. That is perfectly ok! The 3Ps are very adaptable.

3. **Find TIME BUBBLES**
   1. I know this is so hard to do. You have a lot of sick, busy, patients. The floor is always crazy. There are 18 patients waiting to be admitted or discharged and all at the same time. Physicians need to be called or are interrupting you to give you verbal orders. Families have questions! Your orientee is so slow!!! I know and I completely understand. I have been there too. My orientee has their head buried in their report sheet and my brain and my heels are already 10 miles ahead of them. And I have to survey the room and then hold on to the chair to prevent myself from getting up until they are ready.

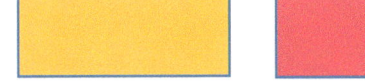

2. Take just 5 minutes when you can. Break the pieces up into small do-able Time Bubbles. I wish we had an hour to prep the day and debrief at the end of the day. But that is a distant memory from my caveman nursing school days, and I know it is not like that anymore. Would be nice though. Instead, we can find Time Bubbles – 5 minutes here and there to pull into a corner and review – the Plan, the Priorities, the Panic Button, a procedure, a medication. *Breaking it into Time Bubbles also avoids information overload to your orientee.*

3. Start with a quick review your preceptor training plan – even if it is only one day. Let them know how you organize your precepting and what to expect. I always start with a quick introduction to each other – and it gives me a quick insight to their previous clinical experience – which is very handy in determining my pace, what I need to explain and how much freedom I give them.

4. **At first, this may take you some additional time to learn and teach it to your orientee.**
   1. Do it every day.
   2. Start with discussing about 1 patient. As you get faster, review all of them.
   3. You WILL GET BETTER.
   4. You WILL GET FASTER.
   5. You WILL GET INTUITIVE about it.
   6. YOU WILL!

5. **PRAISE QUESTIONS! I love questions! I love to let them talk things through out loud.** It shows the wheels are turning. Questions are fantastic! *Preceptors need to love questions!* How many ways are you prepared to teach the same topic? I believe we need to have 3-5 different ways ready to teach things. People are different learners. Fear and Stun affect learning. Experience affects learning. Be ready for questions and abundant with the praise – especially for questions!

6. **The PRECEPTOR TAKES THE LEAD IN CLINICAL EMERGENCIES. YOU are the experienced Nightingale.**
    1. Quickly assess how much you need to take over or can you use The 3Ps right then and there,
    2. Talk out loud, if you can, about what you are doing, why you are doing it, what the priorities are and, your preparation for emergencies.
    3. Stay with them – you will always see more than they will.
    4. Gradually let them take the lead – with you in the passenger seat – ready with praise, questions, support or the emergency brake!

7. **Debrief during or after the shift.** Immediate feedback is critical to connecting the learning dots. Don't wait until the next shift or an evaluation to give feedback.

    And really, don't wait until the evaluation. Use your Time Bubbles. Otherwise, it is not only unfair, it handicaps learning because the memory has faded. If you only have the orientee for one shift or a few hours, there may not be another opportunity to share your wisdom and feedback.

8. **Give them some feedback, some praise and a pearl.** Take the 5 -10 minutes, even as you are walking out the door. They are dying to know what you thought. And you already have 20 things in your head you want to review. You both need it. Just give it 10.

The 3Ps Exercises

In the following pages are exercises for each part of The 3Ps Plan.
Each section is followed by a page for your own notes.

Feel free to make copies.
Use them in your daily precepting.
Write your own Practice scenarios.
Write notes.
Add your own ideas.
Make your precepting experience spectacular!!

H. The 3Ps Handout

Print them out and share!

 ## Plan

THE PLAN:

1. Start with this piece at the beginning of your day
2. This is the list of 1000 things to do you heard in Report (Shift Report, Admission Report, Transfer Report or the mob that met you at the door when you came in the office
3. You are gathering all the information you need, here.
4. Don't worry about getting it all done. Just write it down.
5. Go to the next step: P/Priorities

 ## Priorities

THE PRIORITIES:

1. Out of the 1000 Things To Do you identified in The Plan, now, choose the TOP 3-5 things that MUST be done as a CLINICAL PRIORITY for your shift or the time you have left with the patient or, your office
2. Start with the CLINICAL PRIORITY

 ## Panic Button

THE PANIC BUTTON:

1. What is the WORST thing that could happen to this patient today?
2. How would you recognize it?
3. What would you do about it?
4. What Resources would you need? Know where they are or pull them together NOW.
5. Who could you Alert to be on watch with you?

Work on being able to discuss all 3Ps AFTER report and BEFORE you start seeing patients.

NOTES

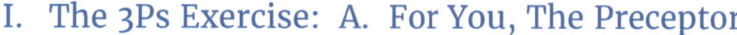

I. The 3Ps Exercise: A. For You, The Preceptor

Preceptors: Try this template for using The 3Ps in your precepting practice. You can use this for BROAD planning: the entire shift or, very SPECIFIC: a procedure, an admission, a diagnosis type. Try it in all four areas! Try to discuss this before you go into a patient room if possible.

P | Plan

1. .Are you Broad (the entire shift) or Specific (a procedure, an admission, a diagnosis type) today: Write down some notes

P | Priorities

1. What are the top priorities you see for your Plan today? Write some notes:
   a.

   b.

   c.

P | Panic Button

1. What is the Panic Button YOU see as the worst thing today? How would you know it was coming or was happening?

2. What preparation and steps would you take? What resources do you want? Who could be their safety buddy?

3. What do you want to discuss about this with your student or orientee?

NOTES

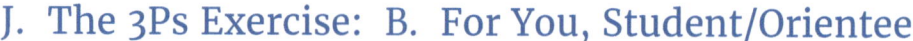

J. The 3Ps Exercise: B. For You, Student/Orientee

Try this template for using The 3Ps in your practice. You can use this for BROAD planning: the entire shift or, very SPECIFIC: a procedure, an admission, a diagnosis type. Try it in all four areas! Make some notes to discuss with your preceptor today or save for later.

P | Plan

1. Are you Broad (the entire shift) or Specific (a procedure, an admission, a diagnosis type) today: Write down some notes

P | Priorities

1. What are the top priorities you see for your Plan today? Write some notes:

    a.

    b.

    c.

P | Panic Button

1. What is the Panic Button you see as the worst thing today? How WOULD you know it was coming or was happening?

2. What preparation and steps would you take? What resources do you want? Who could be your safety buddy?

3. What questions do you have that we can help you with?

NOTES

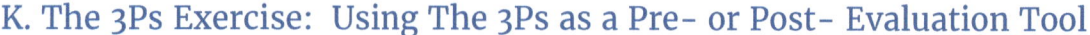

K. The 3Ps Exercise: Using The 3Ps as a Pre- or Post- Evaluation Tool

This is a great tool to easily and quickly get both an overview and detailed look at how your orientee – or yourself – are doing. I have used this each time I first meet an orientee, as a guide as we go along and as I consider my final evaluation.

P Plan

1. Can they identify a list of things to do for the shift?
2. Can they identify a sequence of things to do for a procedure, admission or diagnosis?
3. Can they identify a list of things to do for each patient?
4. What is their report style?
    a. Can they receive nursing report and then tell you The 3Ps?
    b. Can they give an effective report?

P Priorities

1. Can they identify the top 3 priorities for the shift no matter how many patients they have?
2. Can they identify the top 3 priorities for each patient?
3. Can they adjust their priorities as the shift progress, a new admission comes or a patient changes status? The 3Ps is a great tool to help them resume their plan.

P Panic Button

1. What is their response to a quickly decompensating status: Action or Stun?
2. Can they predict a few variables of 'worse case scenarios'?
3. Do they recover a Stun response with your direction?
4. Do you see them incorporating learning experiences and knowledge to improve with the next situation?
5. Does each experience with an emergency improve?
6. Are they engaging, asking questions, helping other staff or quiet and isolative?

NOTES

K. The 3Ps Exercise: Where Else Can You Use The 3Ps? Everywhere!

Here are some of the ways I have used The 3Ps at work ... and at home! Nurses are masters of the multi-task! Our critical-thinking skills don't stop when we leave work, do they? They are good for staff, students – spouses, kids and ... well... everywhere!

- A quick evaluation, plan and action for an orientee I only have for one day.

- An orientee is brought to me having trouble in orientation. This is my own way to see and hear with my own eyes, and evaluate their status – and their potential and plan their success.

- As Preceptor Mama to all my graduated orientees and other post-orientation nurses when they ask me questions.

- When I assist new nurses in new situations.

- Presenting a "Bedside Campfire" case presentation to new staff, orientees and students

- Presenting my evaluation of an orientee to a charge nurse or Director.

- Assisting myself in a new acute patient situation – i.e. learning CVVH with a vented patient and multiple hemodynamic intravenous drips.

- Transitioning from an ICU staff position to a cardiology triage staff position.

- Teaching the kids study skills for school.

- Managing a kid with a newly casted broken arm and a new laundry room flood.

M. Practice Scenarios

As an experienced preceptor and nurse, you have a treasure chest full of experiences – good and bad, easy and hard and those that changed the course of your career.

Dig into that treasure chest and use your own experiences to design some Practice Scenarios that will help you teach The 3Ps.

Use your own experiences.
Use experiences you have seen on your unit.
Use pieces of experiences and create your own scenarios.
Consider the teaching concept you want to cover and design a scenario with The 3Ps.

Write your notes here...

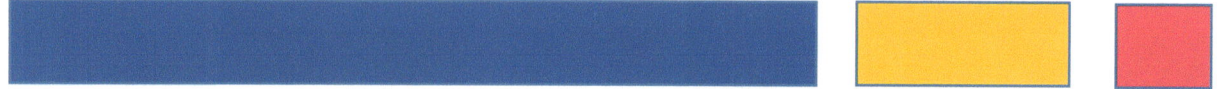

M. PRACTICE SCENARIOS

A. SCENARIO 1

3Ps Focus

Description

M. PRACTICE SCENARIOS

B. SCENARIO 2

3Ps Focus

Description

M. PRACTICE SCENARIOS

C. SCENARIO 3

3Ps Focus

Description

M. PRACTICE SCENARIOS
  D. SCENARIO 4

3Ps Focus

Description

N. Appendix – Handouts

Please see the following pages for printable formats of all the diagrams and exercises I have discussed in this eBook. Please feel free to make as many copies as you like to use during your precepting or orientation experience! I hope they are helpful!

A. The 3Ps Handout
B. The 3Ps Exercise: For the Preceptor/Mentor
C. The 3Ps Exercise: For the Student
D. The 3Ps Exercise: Using The 3Ps as a Pre or Post Evaluation
E. The 3Ps Exercise: Create Your Own Practice Scenarios

A.   The 3Ps Handout

Work on being able to discuss all 3Ps after report and before you start seeing patients.

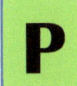 ## Plan

THE PLAN:
1. Start with this piece at the beginning of your day
2. This is the list of 1000 things to do you heard in Report (Shift Report, Admission Report, Transfer Report or the mob that met you at the door when you came in the office
3. You are gathering all the information you need, here.
4. Don't worry about getting it all done. Just write it down.
5. Go to the next step: P/Priorities

 ## Priorities

THE PRIORITIES:
1. Out of the 1000 Things To Do you identified in The Plan, now, choose the TOP 3-5 things that MUST be done as a CLINICAL PRIORITY for your shift or the time you have left with the patient or, your office
2. Start with the CLINICAL PRIORITY

 ## Panic Button

THE PANIC BUTTON:
1. What is the WORST thing that could happen to this patient today?
2. How would you recognize it?
3. What would you do about it?
4. What Resources would you need? Know where they are or pull them together NOW.
5. Who could you Alert to be on watch with you?

The 3Ps Exercise: B. For You, The Preceptor

Preceptors: Try this template for using The 3Ps in your precepting practice. You can use this for BROAD planning: the entire shift or, very SPECIFIC: a procedure, an admission, a diagnosis type. Try it in all four areas! Try to discuss this before you go into a patient room if possible.

 ## Plan

1. Are you Broad (the entire shift) or Specific (a procedure, an admission, a diagnosis type) today: Write down some notes

Priorities

1. What are the top priorities YOU see for your Plan today? Write some notes:

    a.

    b.

    c.

Panic Button

1. What is the Panic Button YOU see as the worst thing today? How would you know it was coming or was happening?

2. What preparation and steps would you take? What resources do you want? Who could be their safety buddy?

3. What do you want to discuss about this with your student or orientee

The 3Ps Exercise: C. For You, Student/Orientee

Try this template for using The 3Ps in your practice. You can use this for BROAD planning: the entire shift or, very SPECIFIC: a procedure, an admission, a diagnosis type. Try it in all four areas! Make some notes to discuss with your preceptor today or save for later.

P | # Plan

1. Are you Broad (the entire shift) or Specific (a procedure, an admission, a diagnosis type) today: Write down some notes

P | # Priorities

1. What are the top priorities you see for your Plan today? Write some notes:

   a.

   b.

   c.

P | # Panic Button

1. What is the Panic Button you see as the worst thing today? How would you know it was coming or was happening?

2. What preparation and steps would you take? What resources do you want? Who could be your safety buddy?

3. What questions do you have that we can help you with?

The 3Ps Exercise: D. Using The 3Ps as a Pre- or Post- Evaluation Tool

This is a great tool to easily and quickly get both an overview and detailed look at how your orientee – or yourself – are doing. I have used this each time I first meet an orientee, as a guide as we go along and as I consider my final evaluation.

 Plan

1. Can they identify a list of things to do for the shift?
2. Can they identify a sequence of things to do for a procedure, admission or diagnosis?
3. Can they identify a list of things to do for each patient?
4. What is their report style?
    a. Can they receive nursing report and then tell you The 3Ps ©?
    b. Can they give an effective report?
    c.

 Priorities

1. Can they identify the top 3 priorities for the shift no matter how many patients they have?
2. Can they identify the top 3 priorities for each patient?
3. Can they adjust their priorities as the shift progress, a new admission comes or a patient changes status? The 3Ps © is a great tool to help them resume their plan.

P **Panic Button**

1. What is their response to a quickly decompensating status: Action or Stun?
2. Can they predict a few variables of 'worse case scenarios'?
3. Do they recover a Stun response with your direction?
4. Do you see them incorporating learning experiences and knowledge to improve with the next situation?
5. Does each experience with an emergency improve?
6. Are they engaging, asking questions, helping other staff or quiet and isolative?

The 3Ps Exercise: E: Practice Scenarios

As an experienced preceptor and nurse, you have a treasure chest full of experiences – good and bad, easy and hard and those that changed the course of your career.

Dig into that treasure chest and use your own experiences to design some Practice Scenarios that will help you teach The 3Ps.

Use your own experiences.
Use experiences you have seen on your unit.
Use pieces of experiences and create your own scenarios.
Consider the teaching concept you want to cover and design a scenario with The 3Ps.

Write your notes here...

3PS FOCUS

SCENARIO DESCRIPTION

M. Join Me for More Exciting Things!

Dear Nightingales and Friends,

I hope you found the 3Ps helpful in your precepting practice and your professional nursing practice!
I hope you will continue to join me in my other Nursing Wit and Wisdom projects!

My vision for Nursing Wit and Wisdom is to "*help nurses and nursing students find ways to stay excited about nursing and understand their unique position to influence others so that they can be inspired about the impact they can make on their patients, families, community and each other.*"

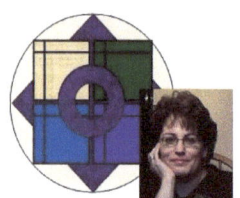

Currently Nursing Wit and Wisdom is an online blog with commentary, education, resources and helpful and creative downloads about everything from learning about IV drips to giving support and feedback to orientees and colleagues. I love writing about my experiences as a nurse and sharing favorite tips and strategies I have learned as a nurse and created as a preceptor and educator. Come visit and sign up for newsletters and blog posts. I will love to see you there!

www.NursingWitAndWisdom.com

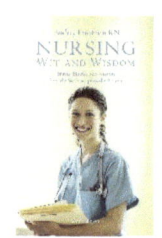

Nursing Wit and Wisdom can also be found in a fun page-turning gift book, "Nursing Wit and Wisdom: Truths, Humor and Wisdom from the Stethescope to the Bedside, 2nd edition". It is full of truths, wisdoms and fun from my own experiences and many great nurses I have had the pleasure and honor of working with. It is available on Amazon and Kindle.

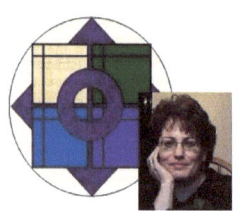

Nursing Wit and Wisdom has also been on Facebook for the last few years. We have over 9000 followers from all over the world. It is exciting to be able to communicate with nurses around the world! Join us for encouragement, support, resources and conversation!

www.Facebook.com/nursingwitandwisdom

I look forward to seeing you somewhere at Nursing Wit and Wisdom!
Inspire and Be Inspired, Nightingales!

Audrey Friedman, RN

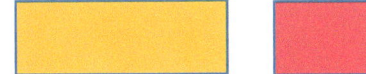

References

Benner, PhD, Patricia.; From Novice to Expert: Excellence and Power in Clinical Nursing Practice; Prentice Hall, 1984, 2001;

Benner, PhD, Patricia: www.nursing-theory.org/theories-ad-models/from-novice-to-expert.php

Sigma Theta Tau International and the International Council of Nurses; Coaching in Nursing;
   https://www.nursingknowledge.org/coaching-in-nursing-oline-course.html

Inspire and Be Inspired Nightingales!

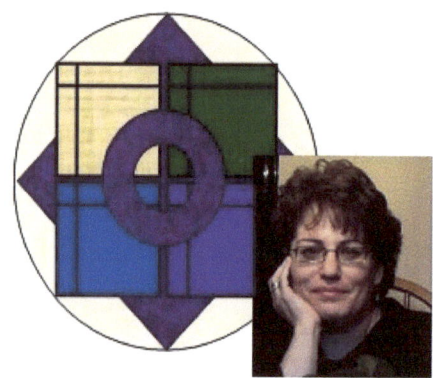

Audrey Friedman, RN